Yoga

Beginners illustrated Poses, Weight Loss

Relieve Stress and Yoga diet

A guide to happy & healthy life

By: Dr.Rogena Saladin

ISBN: 9781795356299
Imprint: Independently published

Copyright © 2019 Rogena, all rights reserved

Contents

Introduction

'**Y**oga' is a Sanskrit expression signifying 'to join, join together or burden together', and the basic reason for yoga is to unite body, psyche, and soul into an agreeable entirety.

The focal strategies for yoga are physical stances or 'asanas' and development, breathing procedures or 'pranayama' and contemplation. Yoga incorporates direction on the sound way of life, dietary patterns, mental demeanor, and Ayurvedic medication is additionally part of the Yogic way to wellbeing and parity.

Hatha yoga is the way of physical yoga, which is the most mainstream part of yoga in the West. 'HA' signifies 'SUN', and 'THA', 'MOON', so Hatha Yoga is the joining, or the burdening together of these diverse energies in agreeable balance, positive and negative, dynamic and responsive.

The origins of yoga

Starting in the old East, yoga has increased huge fame in the advanced western world. Its picture has advanced from those photographs we may have seen of the remarkable routine with regards to inconceivably adaptable cotton-clad religious zealots in India or the seventies side interest of hippy types! Yoga has moved toward becoming a piece of the picked way of life of thousands of westerners looking for some genuine equalization, wellbeing, and prosperity in their lives. Encounters of yoga can be near nature, out of entryways or on the rough ground in substantial tents with somewhat slippy covers on summer withdraws or at celebrations. Be that as it may, it is likewise regular presently to see the brilliantly serene and very much prepared yoga studios in the towns and urban communities as well.

Yoga educators appear to be perhaps significantly cooler than DJs nowadays, making their own tracks by bike, bike, or nippy Mini through city avenues starting with one class then onto the next, taking life at their very own picked pace, holidaying in staggering spots, showing the much-refreshing strategies and standards of yoga to appreciative and excited city inhabitants.

There are yoga magazines, beautiful yoga occasions and a rainbow of extraordinary yoga pack you can purchase. Yet, regardless of anything else, all you truly need to profit by the old knowledge of yoga is your very own body, psyche and soul, some self-restraint, and a not too bad educator to kick you off.

Chapter 1

Beginners illustrated Poses

1. Mountain Pose

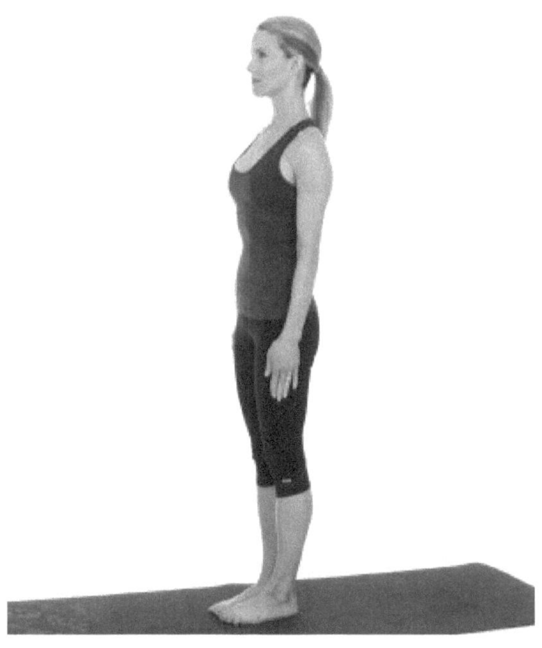

Stand tall with feet together, shoulders lose, weight
uniformly dispersed through your bottoms, arms at sides.

Take a whole breath and raise your hands overhead, palms confronting each other with arms straight. Rise up toward the sky with your fingertips.

2. Downward Facing Dog

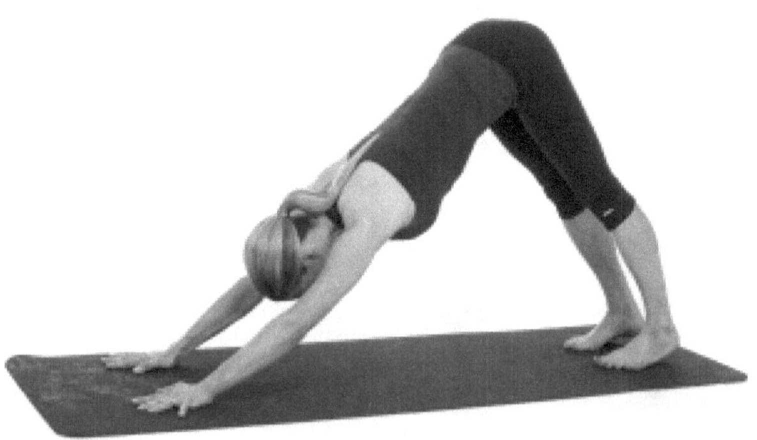

Begin each of the fours with hands straightforwardly under shoulders, knees under hips.

Walk hands a couple of crawls forward and spread fingers wide, squeezing palms into the tangle.

Twist toes under and gradually squeezes hips toward the roof, bringing your body into an upset V, squeezing shoulders from ears. Feet ought to be hip-width alone, knees marginally bowed.

Hold for 3 full breaths.

3. Warrior

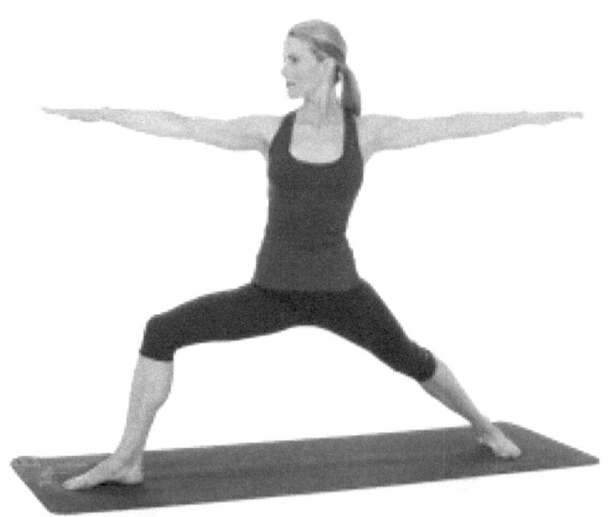

Remain with legs 3 to 4 feet separated, turning right foot out 90 degrees and left a foot in marginally.

Convey your hands to your hips and loosen up your shoulders, at that point stretch out arms out to the sides, palms down.

Curve right knee 90 degrees, keeping knee over lower leg; look out over the correct hand. Remain for 1 minute.

Switch sides and rehash.

4. Tree

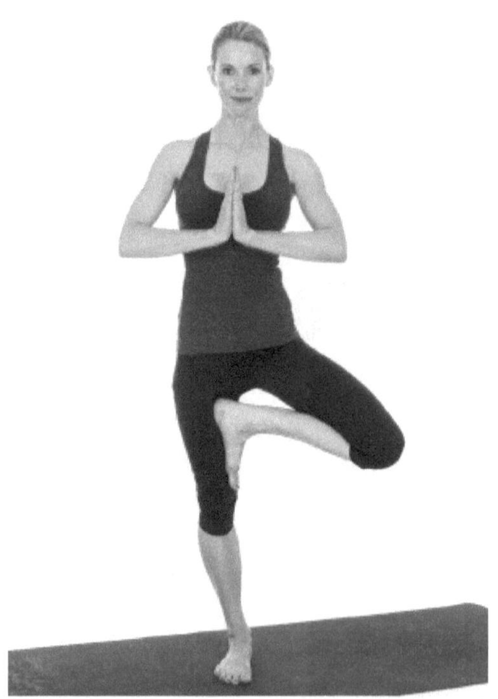

Remain with arms at sides.

Move weight onto left leg and place the underside of the correct foot inside left thigh, keeping hips looking ahead.

When adjusted, get hands in front of you in supplication position, palms together.

On an inward breath, broaden arms over shoulders, palms isolated and confronting each another. Remain for 30 seconds.

Lower and rehash on inverse side.

Make it simpler: Bring your correct foot to within your left lower leg, keeping your toes on the floor for equalization. As you show signs of improving balance, move your foot to within your left calf.

5. Bridge Pose

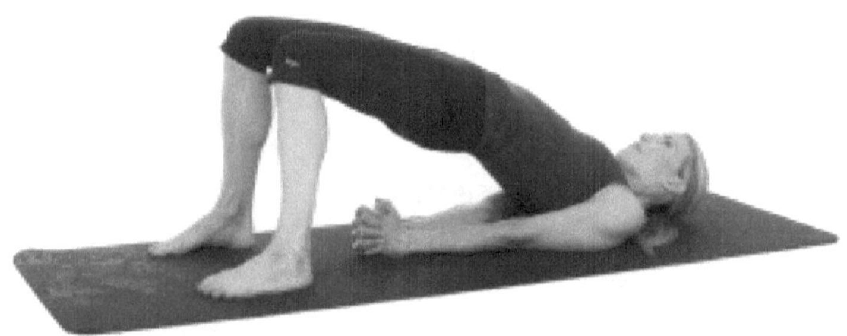

Stretches chest and thighs; broadens the spine

Lie on the floor with knees twisted and straightforwardly over heels.

Place arms at sides, palms down. Breathe out; at that point squeeze feet into floor as you elevate hips.

Fasten hands under lower back and squeeze arms down, lifting hips until the point that thighs are parallel to the floor, bringing chest toward the button. Hold for 1 minute.

Make it less demanding: Place a pile of cushions underneath your tailbone.

6. Triangle

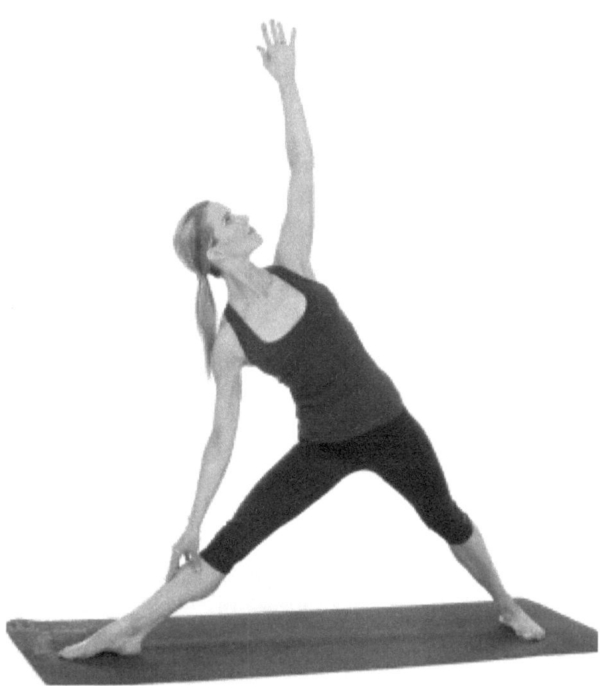

Stretch out arms out to sides, by then contort around your correct leg.

Stay with feet around 3 feet isolated, toes on your correct foot swung out to 90 degrees, left foot to 45 degrees.

Enable your correct hand to contact the floor or lay on your correct leg underneath or over the knee, and broaden the fingertips of your left hand toward the roof.

Turn your look toward the rooftop, and hold for 5 breaths.

Stand and rehash on inverse side.

7. Seated Twist

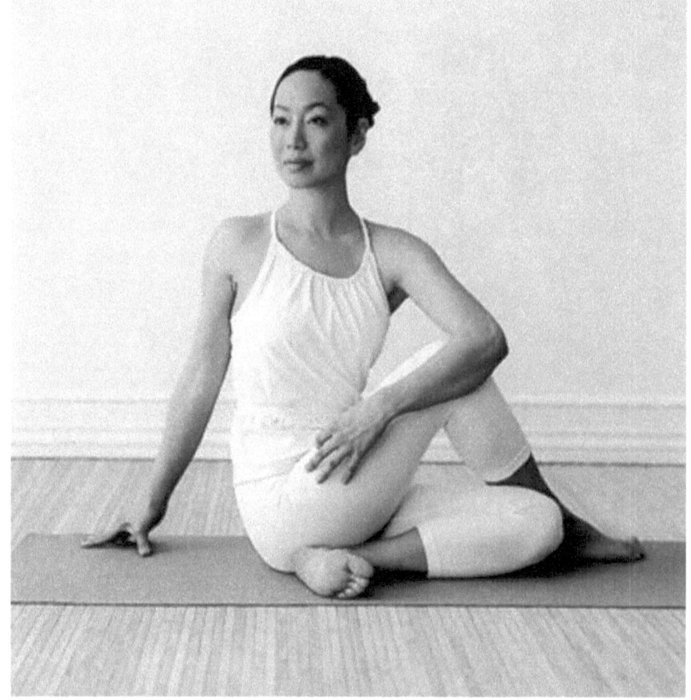

Stretches shoulders, hips, and back; builds dissemination; tones belly; reinforces obliques

Sit on the floor with your legs broadened.

Traverse outside of left thigh; twist a left knee. Keep right knee indicated the roof.

Put a left elbow to the outside of right knee and right hand on the floor behind you.

Wind all right as you can, moving from your guts; keep the two sides of your butt on the floor. Remain for 1 minute.

Switch sides and rehash.

Make it less demanding: Keep base leg straight and place two hands on raised knee. In the event that your lower back rounds forward, sit on a collapsed cover.

8. Cobra

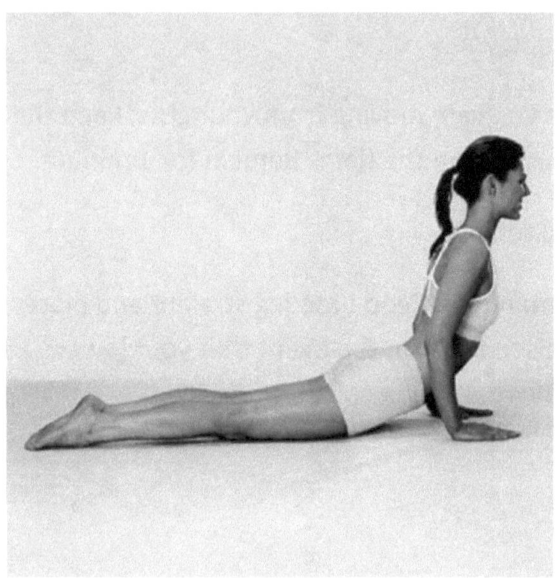

Lie face down on the floor with thumbs explicitly under shoulders, legs stretched out with the highest points of your feet on the floor.

Fix your pelvic floor, and tuck hips descending as you press your gluts.

Press bears down and far from ears.

Push through your thumbs and pointers as you raise your chest toward the divider before you.

Unwind and rehash.

9. Pigeon Pose

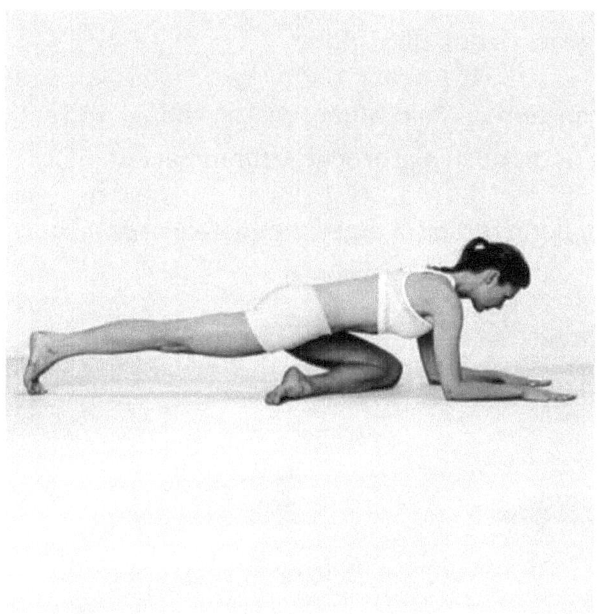

Focuses on the pisiforms (a profound gluteal muscle)

Start in a full push-up position, palms adjusted under shoulders.

Place left knee on the floor close shoulder with left heel by right hip.

Drop down to lower arms and carry right leg down with the highest point of the foot on the floor (not appeared).

Keep chest lifted to the divider before you, looking down.

In case you're progressively adaptable, convey chest down to the floor and broaden arms before you.

Draw navel in toward the spine and fix your pelvic-floor muscles; contract right half of gluts.

Twist right toes under while squeezing the chunk of the foot into the floor, pushing through your impact point.

Twist knee to floor and discharge; complete 5 reps all out, at that point switch sides and rehash.

10. Crow Pose

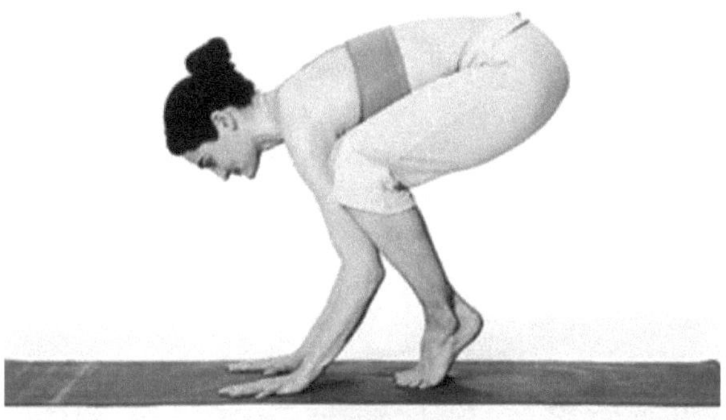

Get into descending puppy position (palms squeezed into tangle, feet hip-width separated) and walk feet forward until the point that knees contact your arms.

Twist your elbows, lift heels off the floor, and lean knees against the outside of your upper arms. Keep toes on the floor, abs drew in and legs squeezed against arms. Hold for 5 to 10 breaths.

Chapter 2

Yoga for weight loss

The act of yoga underpins physical, mental, and otherworldly advancement that enables you to make the best form of yourself.

Yoga may likewise be a powerful device to enable you to get in shape, particularly the more dynamic types of yoga. What's more, you may find that the mindfulness increased through a delicate, loosening up yoga practice causes you to get in shape too.

Numerous specialists concur that yoga works in various approaches to realize a sound weight. How about we investigate a couple of those ways.

Yoga and calorie burning

While yoga isn't generally viewed as an oxygen-consuming activity, there are particular kinds of yoga that are more physical than others.

Dynamic, extreme styles of yoga enable you to consume the most calories. This may help avoid weight gain. Ashtanga, Vinyasa, and power yoga are instances of increasingly physical sorts of yoga.

Vinyasa and power yoga are typically offered at hot yoga studios. These kinds of yoga keep you moving continually, which encourages you to consume calories.

Practicing yoga may in like manner empower you to make muscle tone and improve your digestion.

While remedial yoga isn't a particularly physical sort of yoga, despite everything it helps in weight reduction. One investigation found that therapeutic yoga was powerful in helping overweight ladies to get more fit, including stomach fat.

These discoveries are particularly encouraging for individuals whose body weight may make increasingly incredible types of yoga troublesome.

An audit of concentrates from 2013 found that yoga is a promising method to help with conduct change, weight reduction, and support by consuming calories, increasing care and decreasing pressure. These variables may assist you with reducing nourishment allow and wind up mindful of the impacts of gorging. More inside and out, amazing investigations are expected to develop these discoveries.

How often should you do yoga to lose weight?

Practice yoga as regularly as conceivable so as to get in shape. You can complete a progressively dynamic, serious practice no less than three to five times each week for somewhere around 60 minutes.

On alternate days, offset out your training with an all the more unwinding, delicate class. Hatha, yin, and remedial yoga classes are extraordinary choices.

In case you're a novice, begin gradually and steadily develop your training. This enables you to develop your quality and adaptability and avert wounds. On the off chance that you don't possess energy for a full class on certain days, complete a self-practice for somewhere around 20 minutes. Permit yourself one entire day of rest every week.

Join your yoga practice with exercises, for example, strolling, cycling, or swimming for included cardiovascular advantages.

As a major aspect of your daily schedule, abstain from gauging yourself straightforwardly after a yoga class, particularly if it's a hot yoga class, since you may lose water load amid the class. Rather, gauge yourself in the

meantime every day.

Yoga poses for weight loss

1. Wide-Legged Forward Bend (Prasarita Padottanasana)

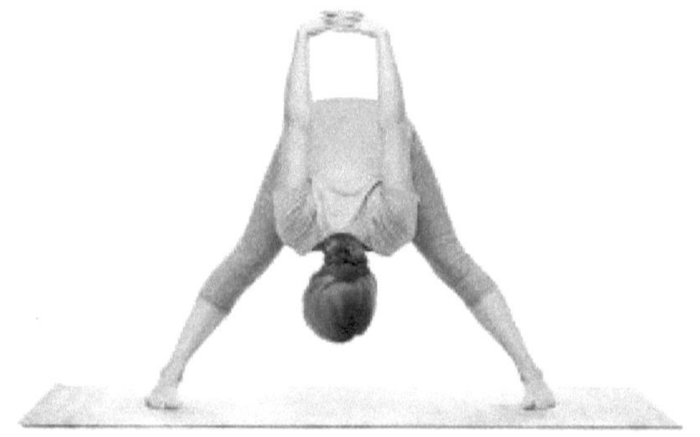

Generally, your hands ought to contact the floor before you in this posture, however, we like the additional shoulder extend!

Spread your feet 3-4 feet isolated, and contort forward at the HIPS, not the midsection. This implies your back ought to be as straight as conceivable when you twist, and you ought not just "hunch" forward.

On the off chance that you're curving fittingly, you will truly feel a strong stretch in the hamstrings. Practice before the mirror to endeavor to get the right frame.

Hold for 5-6 breaths. In the event that you feel great enough, catch the hands behind the back. Attempt to convey them up towards the roof to give the arms and shoulders an additional stretch.

2. Lunge (Anjaneyasana)

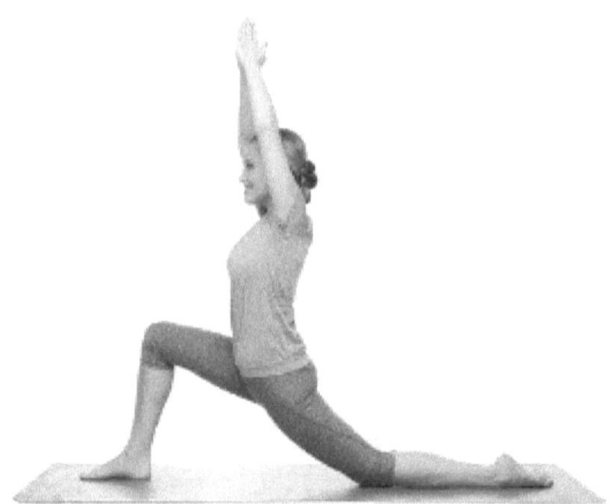

This is a standout amongst the best stances for extending the hips. Numerous individuals will, in general, have tight hips from sitting before a PC throughout the day. It will likewise help increment your adaptability for the parts if that happens to be one of your objectives.

Keep in mind that your hands can be wherever you require them to be in this asana, and their area regularly figures out what muscles you are extending.

On the off chance that you raise the arms up and tilt them in reverse, you will carry this stretch into the back just as the hips. You can in like manner pass on the arms down to your sides and behind you a bit to extend the lower back. The third choice is to lay them on the knee before you, in spite of the fact that you won't get as profound of a stretch in the hips.

Ensure your front knee is as near 90 degrees as could reasonably be expected.

Hold for 30 seconds, and repeat on the contrary side.

3. Half Boat Pose (Ardha Navasana)

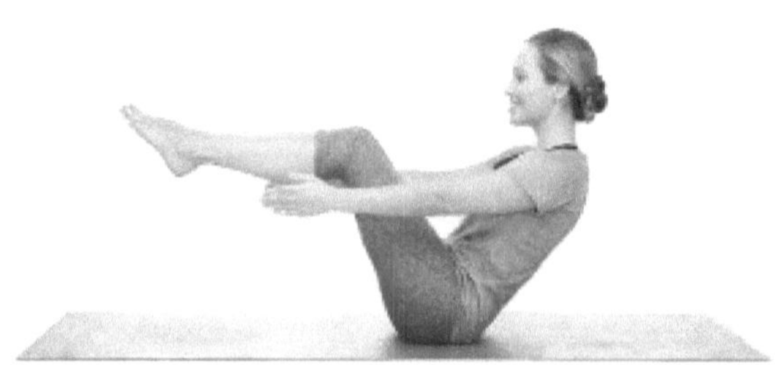

This is a standout amongst the best stances for extending

the hips. Numerous individuals will, in general, have tight

hips from sitting before a PC throughout the day. It will

likewise help increment your adaptability for the parts if

that happens to be one of your objectives. Keep in mind

that your hands can be wherever you require them to be

in this asana, and their area regularly figures out what

muscles you are extending. On the off chance that you

raise the arms up and tilt them in reverse, you will carry

this stretch into the back just as the hips. You can in like manner pass on the arms down to your sides and behind you a bit to extend the lower back. The third choice is to lay them on the knee before you, in spite of the fact that you won't get as profound of a stretch in the hips. Ensure your front knee is as near 90 degrees as could reasonably be expected.

Hold for 30 seconds, and repeat on the contrary side.

4. Side Plank (Vasisthasana)

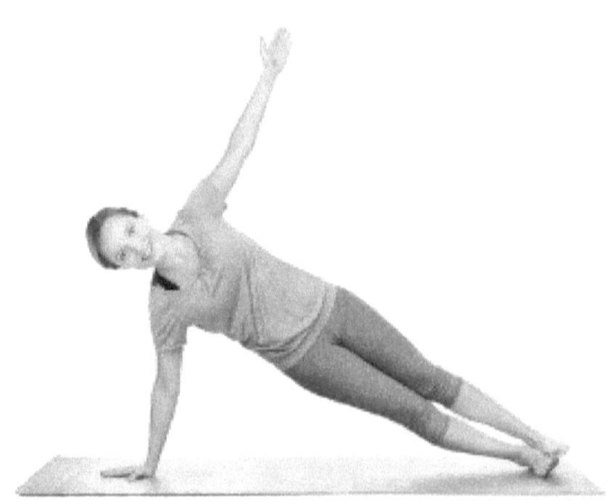

It's no enormous shock that some sort of the "board"

made this summary of yoga asanas for weight reduction.

The board and most of its assortments are staggering for

the abs!

Start in normal board position with your palms look down

on the yoga tangle, bear width separated, and your toes

together on the tangle.

Tilt your feet to the other agree with the objective that the outside right 50% of your right foot is contacting the tangle and the left foot is over the right (as presented previously).

Move your weight onto your correct hand as you expel your left hand from the beginning. Steadily lift your left arm straight up before you towards the rooftop.

Your hips and shoulders should be "stacked" in this stance, implying that they ought to specifically in accordance with one another and not inclining forward or in reverse.

Hold for 30 seconds, and repeat on the contrary side.

5. Tree Pose (Vriksasana)

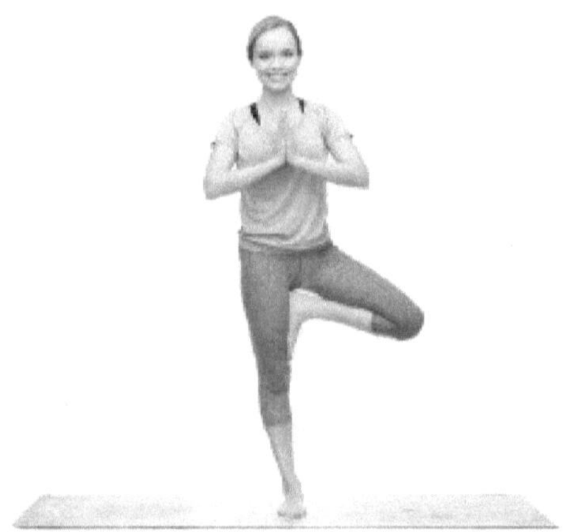

Try not to be tricked by tree present. It's harder to change
in this stance than it looks!

Obtain your left foot to lay inside your left thigh. Keep
your back straight. Your body may tend to slender forward
when attempting to adjust yet bring your shoulders back
up.

Keep your hands squeezed together at your heart to help

with parity, at that point have a go at lifting them over

your head with your hands pointed towards the roof.

Hold for 30 seconds, and repeat on the contrary side.

6. Revolved Lunge Pose (Parivrtta Anjaneyasana)

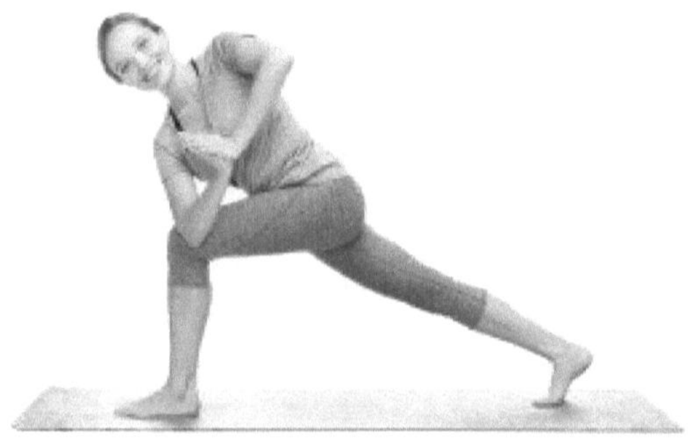

In the event that you have to, keep the correct hand on the floor beside the left foot for help while getting into this posture.

Endeavor to stay your front knee bowed at a 90-degree purpose and your extended leg straight.

Speed up your right elbow to rest your left knee, and join the hands. Press the hands into one another to build the stretch in the back and bears.

Fix your center whereas during this posture for a further exercise within the abs!

Hold for 5-6 breaths or up to thirty seconds, and rehash on the alternative aspect.

7. Chair Pose (Utkatasana)

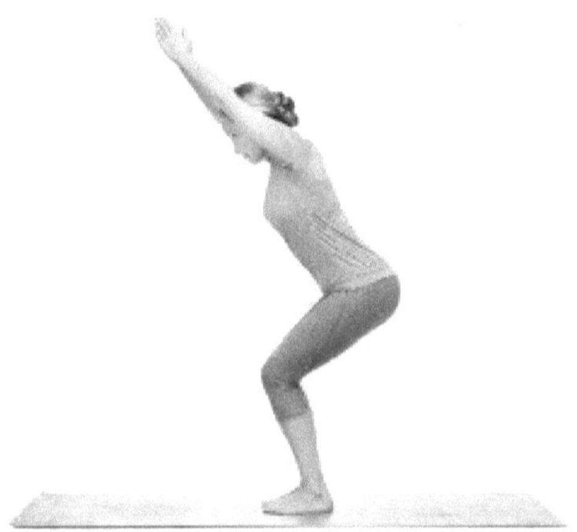

This is the yoga version of a squat hold and conjointly due

to a spot amongst the yoga asanas for weight loss. you'll

feel it in your quad.

Keep the feet along and also the arms straight higher than

you as you lower into a squatting position.

Make sure that you simply will still see your feet before of your knees. If you can't, your knees square measure bent too so much forward.

Try to tuck your hips in slightly, and avoid arcuate the rear an excessive amount of.

Try to get your thighs as about to parallel to the ground as attainable while not compromising your type.

Hold for thirty seconds.

8. Houlderstand (Sarvangasana)

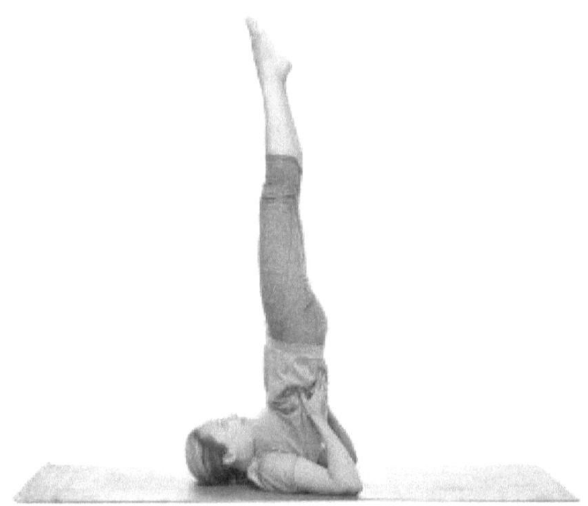

This is thought-about Associate in Nursing inversion as a

result of your body is upper side down! Inversions like an

acrobatic stunt, forearm stand, and gymnastic exercise will

build yoga observe terribly fun! Begin along with your back

on the bottom, your knees slightly bent, and your feet

within the air. Press your hands flat on the bottom, and

use them to roll yourself backward on your higher back.

As you are doing this, bring the hands to your lower back,

simply higher than your hips, to stay yourself upright.

Slowly extend your legs toward the ceiling. Beginner

Modification: If you're having an issue staying up, place

your hands on your hips to assist support your weight

higher.

Hold for 5-6 breaths, and work towards thirty seconds.

Chapter 3

Types of yoga

There are numerous different kinds of yoga out there, whether or not you would like an additional physically hard category or a simple, relaxing, contemplative category. With every vogue a touch completely different from the others, you will find variations betting on the teacher. I like to recommend giving a couple of designs and academics a strive before selecting your favorite.

although you are a seasoned yogi with an obsessive apply, flexibility and variation with any of the subsequent designs may enhance your overall yoga expertise and challenge you to interrupt out of your temperature.

Hatha yoga

The Indo-Aryan term "hatha" is Associate in Nursing umbrella term for all physical postures of yoga. within the West, yoga merely refers to any or all the opposite types of yoga (Ashtanga, Iyengar, etc.) that ar grounded during a physical observe. However, there ar alternative branches of yoga like kriya, raja, and destiny yoga that ar break free the physical-based yoga observe. The physical-based yoga is that the hottest and has various designs. yoga categories ar best for beginners since they're sometimes paced slower than alternative yoga designs. Hatha categories these days ar a classic approach to respiration and exercises. If you're new to yoga, yoga may be a nice entry purpose to the observe.

Iyengar yoga

Iyengar yoga was based by B.K.S. Iyengar and focuses on alignment yet as elaborate and precise movements. In associate degree Iyengar category, students perform a range of postures whereas dominant the breath. Generally, causes ar control for a protracted time whereas adjusting the trivia of the pose. Iyengar depends heavily on props to assist students good their type and go deeper into poses during a safe manner. though you won't jump around, you'll positively get an exercise associate degreed feel improbably open and relaxed when an Iyengar category. This vogue is absolutely nice for individuals with injuries World Health Organization got to work slowly and methodically.

Kundalini yoga

Kundalini yoga observe is equal elements non-secular and physical. This vogue is all concerning emotional the kundalini energy in your body same to be cornered, or coiled, within the lower spine. These categories extremely work your core and respiratory with fast-moving, reviving postures, and respiratory exercises. These categories square measure pretty intense and might involve singing, mantra, and meditation.

Ashtanga yoga

In Sanskritic language, Ashtanga is translated as "Eight Limb path." Ashtanga yoga involves an awfully physically hard sequence of postures, thus this sort of yoga is certainly not for the beginner. It takes associate old yogi to essentially find it irresistible. Ashtanga starts with 5 sun salutation A's and 5 sun salutation B's and so moves into a series of standing and floor postures. In Mysore, India, individuals gather to observe this way of yoga along at their own pace—if you see Mysore-led Ashtanga, it's expected of you to understand the series. Vinyasa yoga stems from Ashtanga because of the flowing vogue linking breath to movement.

Vinyasa yoga

Vinyasa suggests that "to place in an exceedingly special way" and during this case yoga postures. Vinyasa is that the most athletic yoga vogue. Vinyasa was tailored from Ashtanga yoga within the Nineteen Eighties. In Vinyasa categories, the movement is coordinated along with your breath and movement to be due to one cause to a different. many sorts of yoga can even be thought of Vinyasa flows like Ashtanga, power yoga, and prana. Vinyasa designs will vary reckoning on the teacher, and there are many alternative varieties of poses in several sequences. I in person teach AN alignment-based sort of vinyasa and choreograph new flows when however, I additionally wish to hold a number of the poses a small amount longer once warming up.

Bikram yoga

If you're trying to sweat in yoga, this is often the fashion for you. Bikram yoga is called when Bikram Choudhury and options a sequence of set poses during a sauna-like room—typically set to one zero five degrees and forty p.c wetness. The sequence includes a series of twenty-six basic postures, with all performed double.

Jivamukti yoga

Jivamukti was based in 1984 by Sharon Ganon and David Life. Jivamukti is principally vinyasa flow-style categories infused with Hindu religious teachings. A series of chants sometimes open the start of sophistication followed up by a series of poses that align with the 5 tenets of Jivamukti yoga and philosophy. At its core, this vogue emphasizes the affiliation to Earth as a living being, thus most Jivamukti devotees follow their eater philosophy.

Chapter 4

Yoga diet

There's heaps of publicity out there once it involves what to eat. Being environmentally aware of our food decisions appears to be the "in" issue straight away. Farm-raised fish, hormone-free beef, free very chicken, farm-to-table and vegetarian restaurants, organic, gluten-free, macrobiotic—the list goes on!

Many people usually mistake a vegetarian diet for being constant as a Hindooism or yoga diet. however, what will it really mean? what's a Hindooism diet?

Sorting through all the fads, a Hindooism diet follows some pretty straightforward rules. in keeping with my yoga guru Hindu Sivananda, the Hindooism diet ought to

embrace the subsequent things.

A yogic diet should be Sattvic.

In yogistic and Ayurvedic philosophy, there square measure 3 qualities (gunas) of all things in nature: 1) Raja (hot, spicy, fast), 2) Tama (slow, lethargic, bland), and 3) Sattva (purity, harmony). These 3 qualities square measure gift altogether things, however in several amounts, creating one quality dominant.

Rajasic foods square measure hot, bitter, dry, salty, or spicy. They overstimulate the mind and excite the passions. In distinction, tamasic foods square measure bland and embody meat, alcohol, tobacco, garlic, onions, soured foods, and ripe substances.

Sattvic food is that the purest diet, the foremost appropriate one for any serious yoga student. It nourishes the body and maintains a peaceful state. This, in turn, calms and purifies the mind, enabling it to perform at its most potential.

A Sattvic diet can ultimately result in true health; a peaceful mind au fait of a work body, with a balanced flow of energy between them.

Sattvic foods include:

- whole meal bread
- fresh fruit and vegetables
- pure fruit juices
- milk
- butter and cheese
- legumes
- nuts
- seeds
- sprouted seeds
- honey and herb teas

A yogic diet should be vegetarian.

The lion could be a nice meat-eater, and he's known as the king of the jungle. However, no animal will match the elephant, an entire feeder, for pure strength. ~Yogi Bhajan

Fear of super molecule deficiency is that the meat-eaters main objection to a feeder diet. Yet, ironically, meat eaters acquire the worst quality super molecule from their food—the super molecule that's dead or dying.

Animal super molecule contains an excessive amount of acid and alternative toxins to be counteracted by the liver; some are eliminated, however, the remainder is deposited within the joints and tissues, resulting in issues like inflammatory disease and cancer.

Uric acid could be a poisonous substance that additionally makes it more durable to succeed in the upper, clear contemplative state as a result of its associated pain in the neck within the blood.

Meat is additionally among the best sources of steroid alcohol, that contributes to the heart condition, hardening of the arteries, and senility. Meat takes 3 days to meet up with the gastrointestinal system. For optimum health, men have to be compelled to digest food inside twenty-four hours, ladies eighteen hours.

Nuts, dairy farm product, ivied greens, and legumes are choked with high-quality supermolecule. Their main residue is polyose, which is inert and doesn't soil the body. It's promptly assimilable, used by the body quickly and with efficiency.

Take time to fast.

The yogis suggest selecting in some unspecified time in the future hebdomadally to quick. a quick is strict, not permitting something to enter the body. Or, it will embrace water and fruit juices. no matter you decide on, confine mind that the goal of your quick is to purify the body and mind.

For me, once every week is fantastic. I select to quick on Ekadashi, the eleventh day of every lunation, determined by yogis to be Associate in Nursing auspicious day.

Practice ahimsa.

The first of the yoga observances (yamas), gospel or

nonviolent resistance will be applied to the food we tend

to eat. creating environmentally-conscious health

decisions that don't hurt people, animals, or the earth

takes acutely aware awareness.

I accustomed purchase drinking water to remain hydrous

and thought it had been healthier than sports drinks. Once

I started to have faith in all the pollution I used to be

caused by browsing such a large amount of water bottles, I

endowed in an exceedingly refillable glass bottle instead,

that is way a lot of environmentally-conscious.

Keep in mind that tiny, on the face of it insignificant changes within the method you eat and live will have massive implications. Above all, keep in mind that you simply are gods and goddesses, and your body may be a temple! Keep food decisions easy, pure, fresh, and use your best judgment. Your inner yogi is aware of best.

Chapter 5

Benefits of yoga

The External Health

There are units numerous edges the interior body experiences that we will solely feel. However, yoga additionally works on the external body, creating it doable for the U.S. to check the advantages. Read on. you'll be pleasantly stunned by these yoga health edges.

The Emotional Health

Yoga creates a powerful affiliation between the mind and therefore the body, and this enhances your emotional health superbly.

It Makes You Smarter

Twenty minutes of yoga improves the brain's ability to quickly and accurately method info (even a lot of therefore than running does), says a study revealed within the Journal of Physical Activity and Health. "While most exercise offers you an option to either zone in or zone out, yoga encourages you to come to this and concentrate," Zimmerman says. "This aware awareness has been related with structural changes within the brain, together with growth within the anterior cortex, a brain region related to government operations, remembering, and a focus."

You Can Do It in the Nude

Naked yoga classes—in those practitioners disrobe to the buff before down-dogging with fellow practitioners—are shooting up everyplace. Offered as male, female, and coed categories, they are meant to require yoga's love-your-body mantra to ensuing level. Cross-check however one girl overcame her naked-yoga fears, gained some confidence, and shrugged off her alleged "imperfections."

It Seriously Slashes Stress

Anyone WHO has ever settled into children creates is aware of yoga is calming. "The tensing and relaxation of muscles throughout yoga—along with conscious awareness of physical sensations—helps the United States relax," Zimmerman says. That will be one reason why simply eight weeks of daily yoga considerably improves sleep quality in individuals with a sleep disorder, in line with a Harvard University study.

It Protects Your Heart

Your yoga teacher is usually talking regarding "opening your heart" for a reason. "Yoga will scale back high-pressure level, unhealthy sterol, and stress, all risk factors for cardiovascular disease, says Larry Phillips, MD, a medical specialist at the NYU Langone center. And it isn't simply the chilliness factor: performing arts savasana (corpse pose) is related to larger enhancements in pressure level compared to easily lying on the couch, consistent with analysis revealed within the Lancet.

www.ingramcontent.com/pod-product-compliance
Lightning Source LLC
Chambersburg PA
CBHW051233250726
48655CB00006B/2745